YOGA
FOR
Curvy
GIRLS
GUIDE

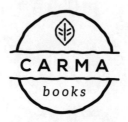

'A conscious approach to health & wellness'

carmabooks.com

You are invited to to join our **Free Book Club**
mailing list. Sign up via our website to receive
special offers and **free for a limited time**
Health & Wellness eBooks!

YOGA

FOR

Curvy

GIRLS

GUIDE

Easy Beginner's
Poses for Women
with Curves

Carmen Reeves

Disclaimer

Your health and wellbeing is important. For that reason, please consult a medical professional before taking part in this, or any other fitness activity. Not all exercises are suitable for everyone, and may result in injury, especially if you already have pre-existing health problems. By taking part in these exercises, you agree to do so at your own risk and assume all associated risk of injury.

Yoga is amazing, and we strongly believe that everyone can benefit from it. However, the information in this book is for informational purposes only, and is not intended to be construed as medical advice, nor should it replace the guidance of a qualified instructor who can guide you personally and tailor a yoga program to your specific requirements.

Bear in mind that there are no 'typical' results from the information provided - as individuals differ, the results will differ. No responsibility is taken for any loss or damage related directly or indirectly to the information in this book. Never disregard professional medical advice or delay in seeking it because of something you have read in this book or in any linked materials.

Carma Books
carmabooks.com

hello@carmabooks.com

CONTENTS

CHAPTER 7

Troubleshooting: Yoga For Period Pain..........78

CHAPTER 8

Troubleshooting: Gentle 5-Minute-Fix Yoga 87

CHAPTER 9

Yoga & The Future: Where To Go From Here ...96

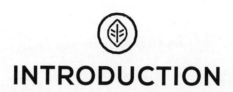

INTRODUCTION

Did you know that over the last few years, a revolution has been gathering place in yoga studios and living rooms of the world? A powerful revolution fronted by women just like you and I who also want to enjoy the massive health and happiness benefits of starting a yoga practice, but because of their body shape have felt too ashamed to even give it a go.

This comprehensive beginner's guide to yoga has been specifically tailored to meet the unique requirements of women just like you and I, *women who are curvy, voluptuous and utterly beautiful*, and would love to enjoy the benefits of yoga but feel nervous, self-conscious or generally uncomfortable about starting.

We deserve to feel and look our best too. We deserve to become more flexible and stronger. And we deserve to be happier, stress-free and feel confident to take on the world with inner vibrancy.

The world would have us believe that to benefit from yoga, you need to have supermodel looks, have a slender physique and be as bendy as a pretzel. But this is simply not true. You only need the desire to learn and a body to practice within to reap yoga's amazing benefits (and I'm pretty sure you have the latter!). There is no better time to start than now, and I will show you how.

I've witnessed the amazing transformative effects of yoga in all of my fellow yogi friends and enthusiasts; I've watched wallflowers blossom into strong, confident and beautiful women, I've seen that inner glow light faces from within, I've seen chronic health conditions heal and stubborn pounds drop off. And I can't wait for these amazing benefits to happen to you.

You see, whilst there's an abundance of information out there on the subject of yoga, very few materials offer help and advice that address our unique needs and concerns.

'Will I ever be able to touch my toes?'

'Do I just look silly?' and;

'Will I ever be able to keep up?'

Let's face it; yoga may pose a little more challenging for us curvier girls. But with my expert advice and practice, you will see how you can achieve fantastic results just like anyone else. I have helped empower curvier women to start a yoga practice no matter what their challenges, or how scared they might feel, and now I'm here to do exactly the same for you.

This book will share with you everything you'll need to know to incorporate yoga into your life from this very moment, avoiding much of the technical jargon that can seem confusing and off-putting, and showing you those all-important tweaks that will assist you through your physical challenges. And at the end of your journey through this book, you will learn how to find a brilliant instructor who will understand your unique challenges and help you continue your yoga journey.

Whether you want to shift a few extra pounds, relieve stress or anxiety, boost your strength and flexibility, look healthier and happier, or even find inner peace - yoga is your answer. **For me, yoga was life changing.** Expect to see wonderful, incredible and surprising changes in your own life.

Yoga really is for every *body*.

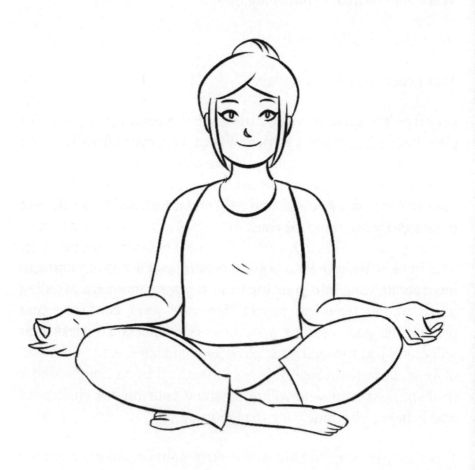

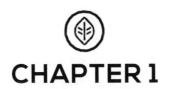

CHAPTER 1

Yoga 101:

Everything You Need To Know

Although it can be really tempting to just get started with the movements to improve your life as quickly as possible, it really is vital to understand some of the history and philosophy of yoga. You see, yoga is about so much more than just physical movement, and to limit our focus to just bending our bodies into the right shapes would be doing it an incredible disservice.

This chapter will give you all of the essential info that will give you a vital head-start, that will help you get results sooner, and progress faster in your journey. You'll learn what yoga really is, understand the essentials about the different styles of yoga and also learn a little about the underlying philosophy and the top benefits that yoga can offer to your body and mind. But don't worry - I'll keep it as beginner-friendly and jargon-free as I possibly can.

Let's take a look.

What is Yoga?

This is probably the hardest question in the world to answer. At its core, it's a movement practice, which originates from India around 3,000 years ago, incorporating various Hindu traditions and practices with a hefty dose of spiritualism.

You might have noticed that yoga has shot up in popularity over the past couple of decades, and this has happened for great reason. **It's part physical therapy and part meditation.** Not only does it get your body feeling strong and healthy (and resurrects that childhood dream of doing the splits!) it also allows you to feel relaxed, alleviates stress, and helps you discover a place of inner peace - to understand the true nature of the world and realize what really matters to you.

Interesting fact: Yoga was originally invented by yogis who found their muscles became stiff and sore after sitting in meditation for long periods of time.

Styles of Yoga

It might surprise you to know that there isn't just one type of yoga, but several subtypes, which have evolved over the history of yoga; each of which best suit different types of people and different needs. As a beginner, it's best to experiment with different styles until you find the perfect fit for you. Let's take a quick look at what these are.

Hatha Yoga

When people talk about yoga, this is usually the one they mean. Most modern classes are commonly based on *Hatha* yoga if not stated otherwise. It's the calm, physically focused style that looks like stretching, whilst also paying attention to the breath.

Each individual pose is treated completely separate, so there is no need to flow through the movements nor keep up with a fast-paced routine.

Overall, it's the best style for calm and relaxation in addition to boosting flexibility, strength and overall wellbeing - and is my personal favorite. *Bikram* and *Ashtanga* yoga are based on this style.

Vinyasa Yoga (aka Power Yoga)

Power yoga is another popular style of yoga that will keep you moving throughout the entire class, and is perfect for shifting any stubborn pounds. Expect plenty of sun salutations (I'll tell you all about those later) and even the odd headstand or two.

Ashtanga Yoga

Ashtanga yoga is another variation of *Hatha* yoga, which concentrates on fast-paced sequences of movement, alongside perfectly timed breathing. Classes are usually quite intense and will likely leave you out of breath. It promotes healthy circulation, weight loss, and helps create a clear and unperturbed mind.

Bikram Yoga (aka Hot Yoga)

Bikram yoga is a unique yoga technique as it's practiced in a heated environment which is said to warm your muscles, easily facilitate stretching and flexibility, detoxifies the body, and helps shift excess weight. Expect to do a sequence of 26 poses twice with a section of breath work midway through.

Iyengar Yoga

If you have ever experimented with Pilates, ballet or are a fan of precision and alignment, *Iyengar* yoga will be the perfect style for you. Expect to see props like blocks and straps to help you recreate these perfect forms. It can be a highly demanding and strict style, but many people will love it for these exactly qualities.

Kundalini

Kundalini yoga literally means 'coiling snake' and is the most spiritual of the types of yoga mentioned here. It's focused on releasing energy which is believed to be located at the base of the spine, and which moves throughout the body. This is mainly achieved through deep breathing.

Which of these styles sounds most appealing to you? Will it be the calm and centered *Hatha* technique, the sweaty *Bikram* approach, the fast-paced *Iyengar* or *Ashtanga* styles, or the spiritual *Kundalini*? Have fun discovering which of these will be your perfect fit!

The Philosophy of Yoga

If you've ever investigated the philosophy of yoga, it's likely that you've found yourself bogged down in details, feeling overwhelmed and actually deterred from trying out a class or two for yourself. This is a tragedy. Whilst there is no denying that the philosophy of yoga is important, you don't have to understand every inch to get great results. Let me explain all you need to know right now.

Yoga seeks unity. Its purpose is to unite the mind, spirit and body, as well as developing perfect harmony between the three aspects of the human being. It's said that this is achieved by paying attention to eight aspects, known as 'the eight limbs'. These are:

1. Yama *(ethical standards)*

2. Niyama *(self-discipline/standards)*

3. **Asanas *(your yoga practice)***

4. Pranayama *(breathing techniques)*

5. Pratyahara *(sensory deprivation)*

6. Dharana *(concentration)*

7. Dhyana *(meditation)*

8. Samadhi *(pure consciousness)*

As mentioned, this information isn't essential at this stage of your journey, so I won't go into too much more detail here, but it can help to understand where the postures fit into the bigger picture.

The Five Main Principles

These eight limbs were eventually simplified into five principles, which you can use right now to make some amazing changes in your life. They are:

1. ***Proper exercise:*** You need to be active and flexible.

2. ***Proper breathing:*** Correct breathing is essential for life.

3. ***Proper relaxation:*** Quietening the body and mind.

4. ***Proper diet:*** Diet affects both your body and mind. If you want best results from your yoga practice, it is essential to ditch the processed foods and concentrate on 'real foods' instead.

5. ***Proper thinking:*** Letting go of toxic thought processes and fostering healthy ones instead.

If you only remember these five things, you'll be well on your way to unlocking the best possible version of you from within. Bear them in mind as you learn.

The Benefits of Yoga

Yoga is wonderful, as there is absolutely nothing like it in the world. It doesn't only target your muscles and physical body, but also your mind, and also helps you find greater harmony between the two.

Despite beginner's hesitations, yoga is actually the perfect regimen for those looking for a gentle start to exercising (especially for those of us on the curvier side) - it is easy on the joints, easily adaptable to everyone's needs, burns a ton of calories, and you can crank up the difficulty levels when you are feeling more confident and experienced.

Here's just a handful of the benefits yoga can offer:

- Increased flexibility

- Better posture

- Decreased stress-levels

- Greater strength in muscles and joints

- Reduces inflammation

- Better balance

- Develops balance

- Protects your spine

- Improves blood flow

- Boosts your immunity and lymph drainage

- Regulates your adrenal glands

- Relieves symptoms of hormonal imbalance or the menopause

- Makes you feel happier (and beat depression)

- Balances blood sugar

- Improves appetite control

- Helps you to focus

- Beats insomnia and helps you to sleep better

- Provides you a great cardio workout

- Heals your mind

And many more. Yoga really is incredible.

CHAPTER 2

Five Easy Ways To Get The Most From Your Yoga Practice

We've covered the essentials of yoga so far in this book, and I can tell that you're itching to get started. But before we do, I'd like to take the opportunity to share with you some really amazing gems of knowledge that will help to propel your yoga practice from simply average to a whole new level.

By following these tips, you'll find it a whole lot easier to get started, to modify the postures to suit your own needs and requirements, and to really enjoy the best health benefits that you possibly can. This is where you will learn how to overcome any issues you might face to move forward in your journey.

So without further ado, let's look at the five easy ways to make the most of the benefits from your yoga practice.

1. Keep an Eye on Your Expectations

Let's be honest here - yoga *is* challenging, especially if it's been a while since you've last exercised (but so is any other form of exercise). Yoga is one of those pursuits that seems effortless when you watch it, but is much harder when you actually give it a go for yourself. Don't let this deter you - there will still be a ton of simple postures you can practice, and you can take it step by step to achieve your goals.

Don't think this is any different because of your shape or size. We all face both mental and physical challenges which we can gently work though with the help of yoga, and provided we keep pushing ourselves to meet our goals and improve, we *WILL* get there. Just don't expect to run before you can walk.

2. Don't Push Through the Pain!

Yoga should never *EVER* feel painful. It's vital that you listen to your body and go at your own pace, or else you run a significant risk of injury and/or exhaustion, no matter what you think you should be able to achieve (or in a class setting, what those around you are doing).

This is *your* yoga practice, no one else's. Nor are there any prizes for attempting the most advanced of postures. Yoga is about your own personal experience and journey to better health and happiness.

If you feel a pose is too difficult, don't be afraid to use modifications, props or even skip the pose altogether until you have more experience under your belt. *Child's Pose* is a brilliant option for those times you need a breather but don't want to quit.

3. Tackle Your Unique Challenges

There are unique limitations and obstacles that you may face as a curvy girl starting a yoga practice. You'll know what I'm talking about; those bigger bellies, rebellious breasts, thicker thighs, curvy bottoms and strong arms all need to be taken into consideration.

You might find that some yoga poses are rather interesting to attempt when you are curvier. Many of my companion yogis complain that they feel like their breasts are about to suffocate them during certain poses, or that they just can't get their ankles together when attempting standing poses. This is perfectly normal.

Simply find the solution that works best for your particular problem. Why not use props such as **straps, bolsters, pillows, blocks, and chairs,** or even modify poses using a **wall** to lean on for support, or **blankets** to lift your shoulders or add support to the lower back. Using a **yoga mat** can make the experience easier and gentler on your joints, and clothing does not need to be any different than regular, comfortable gym-wear that is light and allows for a full range of motion.

And in case you're wondering - the best solution to that suffocating breast problem is to wear a very supportive sports bra or wear a strap around your body just beneath your armpits. Give it a go!

4. Breathe Properly

It might seem like a no-brainer to hear that you should breathe properly, but a surprising number of us don't, and will never reach our full potential when it comes to health and happiness. When you practice yoga, it's vital that you focus your attention on your breath, as it is a significant part of a yoga practice and will extend and improve the benefits you will experience.

Primarily, this means nothing more complicated that paying attention to your breath, and ensuring that you are filling all parts of your lungs, and exhale through your nose. Don't hold your breath, but just breathe, be present, relax and enjoy the experience of practicing yoga.

5. Concentrate

Yoga is your opportunity to disconnect from everyday life, recharge your batteries and calm and relax your mind. The only way you can achieve this is to focus your attention on your practice itself, and resist the urge to let your mind wander into random thoughts, like what you're going to cook for dinner or whether or not you said the right thing to your co-worker the other day.

Most of us are accustomed to racing thoughts and thinking of around a million things at once, so in the beginning it might be hard to let go and get into '*the zone*'. But after a little practice, you'll soon find that it gets easier and easier, and you actually enjoy the mental 'breathing' space that you create.

A great trick is to focus on the pattern of your breath, and pay attention as you move through the postures. If your mind wanders, simply bring it back to your breath and your movement and start again.

Of course, you *can* whizz through all of the postures and get much fitter and stronger as a result. But if you really want to enjoy the full life-changing benefits of practicing yoga it's worth taking it all very slowly, listening to your body, making the necessary modifications, paying attention to your breath, and also focusing your attention as best you can. All of these things will maximize the positive impact it has on your life, and help you heal inside and out.

Up until now, this book has provided you with everything you need to know about yoga in general, from its history, the varying styles, the philosophy behind it all and even its main health benefits.

But now it's time to get moving! Let's get started with a short yoga program that you can do from absolutely anywhere, and that even the absolute beginner can try.

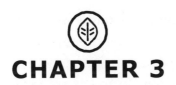

CHAPTER 3

Start Practicing:
Sun Salutations For Yoga Success

We've finally reached the best part of this entire book - the poses, or *asanas*, themselves. You are about to learn the wonderful ways in which you can feel amazing, energize your mind and body, relieve stress, anxiety, period pain, insomnia and those awful days at work. Your health will improve beyond your wildest dreams and you'll start to achieve the kind of happiness you have always wanted.

I understand that this must sound like a bunch of far-fetched claims, but let me assure you that it most certainly isn't. All you need to do is create your own practice based on the postures and sequences you are about to learn, and you will see the results for yourself.

We are going to kick-off with a sequence of Sun Salutations, known in Sanskrit as *surya namaskar*.

Intro to Sun Salutations

In the next chapter, we'll be working through this sun salutation sequence together and exploring the ways in which it can benefit your body. And don't worry - you'll also learn tweaks and modifications to suit your body's needs.

A sun salutation is a specific sequence of yoga postures, *or asanas*, which work effectively together and allow you to 'flow' between one posture to the next in a gentle and fluid way. You could best think of it in terms of yoga 'choreography'. They provide a great foundation for your yoga practice and will help you to understand and unlock the principles so you can enjoy maximum benefits for your mind, body and soul.

Sun salutations are an excellent go-to practice that will help awaken and energize your body, warm up and stretch your muscles and help you prepare for your day. **If you only practice a minimal amount of yoga on a regular basis, make it a sun salutation.** They're generally best practiced earlier on in the day.

Once you have mastered the basics of the sun salutations, and have understood the principles and your personal needs, you can move forwards in your practice to explore more postures - or troubleshoot some of your body issues such as period pain, insomnia, depression and anxiety, daily muscles aches, or even weight loss. You'll find small groups of these additional moves later on in this book.

So, find yourself a quiet place free from distractions, switch off that cell phone, and let's begin!

Mountain Pose
Tadasana

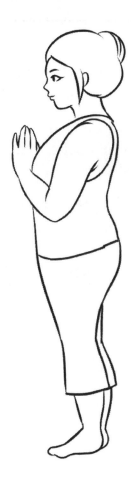

Whilst Mountain Pose offers a ton of benefits like improving your posture, strengthening your thighs, knees, and ankles and relieving sciatica, it's really all about finding your center and your balance. This might sound easy and even a little too simple, but it's actually more challenging than it sounds. After the stresses and strains of everyday life, it can be hard to switch off and regroup your sense. This pose will help you do exactly that.

1. Stand on your mat with your feet firmly on the ground, shoulders pulled back down from your ears, and crown of your head gently pulled towards the sky.

2. Pay attention to your feet and either move them together until they are touching from your big toe right back to your heel, or otherwise placed hip width apart. Make sure they are parallel and facing forward.

3. Place the palms of your hands together and hold them just in front of your chest, thumbs touching your breastbone.

4. Take a deep breath and allow the air fill up your lungs from the very bottom, into your belly, into your chest and right up under your shoulders. Then exhale slowly.

5. Stay in the pose for a further four breaths.

Upward Salute

Urdhva Hastasana

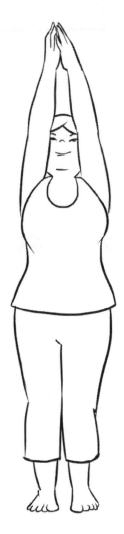

This pose provides the perfect warm-up stretch for your entire body, the kind of stretch that makes you go *"aaah!"* - it feels that good. It's also brilliant for asthma, back ache and fatigue as it helps open up the lungs, extend and nourish the spine and get everything moving as it should in the digestive system. Here's how to do it.

1. From Mountain Pose, keep your shoulders relaxed and away from your ears, and keep grounding down through your feet.

2. Take a deep breath and raise your hands overhead, palms still touching. Reach towards the sky. Don't worry if you're a little tight in the shoulders and your hands won't touch - just keep them parallel and reach as high as you can.

3. Without compressing your neck, tip your head back slightly and gaze upwards. If you find your balance suffers, return to looking directly ahead of you, close your eyes and breathe.

4. Hold for five breaths before moving into the next posture

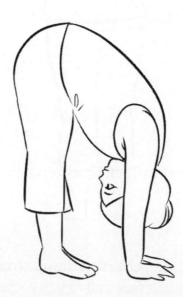

Standing Forward Bend
Uttanasana

This might well be my favorite asana of them all. Again, it looks mighty simple but it can be quite challenging and highly beneficial for your entire body. It's the perfect way to de-stress and help overcome mild depression. As well as stretching those hamstrings and calves, it will also do wonders for any symptoms of menopause, high blood pressure, infertility or headaches and migraines.

1. From Upward Salute, gently lower your hands and rest them lightly upon your hips.

2. Now exhale and fold yourself forward from your hip joints reaching with your hands in front of you. If your belly gets in the way at this point, use your hands to tuck it gently out of the way, widen your legs, and try again. Widen your legs if you need to, but make sure your feet stay parallel.

3. Continue this extension forwards and allow yourself to reach downwards towards your feet instead. Don't get too hung up on touching those toes - that will come in time. Draw in your tummy muscles, and lengthen that torso towards the ground.

4. We will be moving towards getting those legs straight, but for now, bend them as deeply as you need to in order to support the rest of your body.

5. For additional arm support, bring in a pair of blocks and place your hands upon them.

6. Relax your head and neck and allow your head to hang loosely towards the ground. Don't forget to breathe.

7. Hold this pose for five breaths, coming out sooner if you need to.

Low Lunge

Anjaneyasana

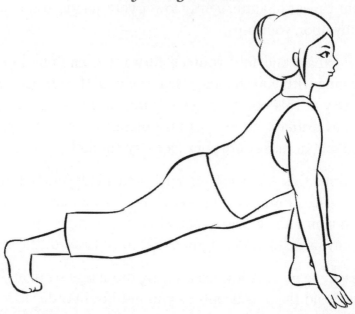

For back problems, sciatica and general aches and pains that can arise, this posture is wonderful. Sink into it to feel a deep stretch through your hips, groin and legs, and warm up your body for the next asanas in the sequence.

1. From Standing Forward Bend, exhale and step back with your left foot. Check in with your right foot and make sure that it is directly under your knee.

2. Keeping your hands on the floor or on any blocks you might be using, press through your palms, spread your fingers wide and use them to help find your stability and balance.

3. Check in with your body, moving your shoulders away from your ears, engaging your stomach muscles and looking directly ahead.

4. Hold the pose for 5 breaths.

Plank Pose

Uttihita Chaturanga Dandasana

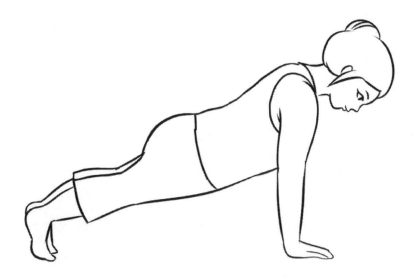

This is another of those poses that looks far easier than it feels. For that reason, build up to the full posture and feel free to modify or use as many props as you like. Don't feel as though you have to push yourself; take it gently and you will soon notice the difference. It's great for strengthening your arms, wrists and spine and will work wonders on your core strength.

1. Starting in Low Lunge with your hands firmly on the floor or on blocks, step back with your right leg so that it joins your left leg behind you.

2. Check in with your body, making sure your wrists are directly under your shoulders and spreading those fingers wide to ensure you have a solid base. Push your shoulder blades down away from your ears.

3. Now lift your thighs upward and lengthen through your spine, keeping your body nice and long and straight. If you find this

challenging, feel free to lower your knees to the floor, or even rest completely. Don't feel defeated - this pose is meant to be challenging, and the longer you practice, the closer you'll get to doing it!

4. Hold pose for 5 breaths.

Low Plank
Chaturanga

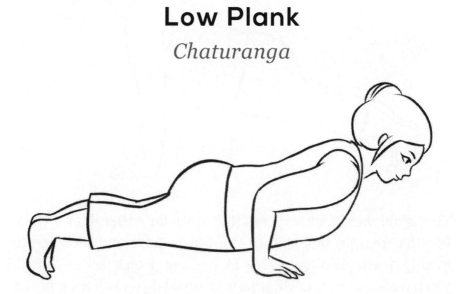

Similar to a high plank, this pose will strengthen your arms, shoulders and leg muscles and works wonders on your core strength and muscle tone in your tummy. It helps prepare your body for more advanced moves and improves your balance and self-esteem at the same time. Sound good? Here's how to do it.

1. Starting from the Plank Pose, bend at the elbows, push your shoulders slightly forward and move your weight forward onto the balls of your feet.

2. Engage your stomach muscles, reach your breastbone forward and create a firm line from your shoulders to your feet.

3. Then lower yourself towards the floor until you are about 6 inches away, maintaining a strong back.

4. Don't panic if you find this pose especially challenging - that's how it's meant to be. You can modify the pose by placing your knees on the floor, widening those arms, or evening coming down onto your forearms instead. If you are still finding it challenging, consider skipping this pose altogether and resting back into Child's Pose.

The Cobra Pose

Bhujangasana

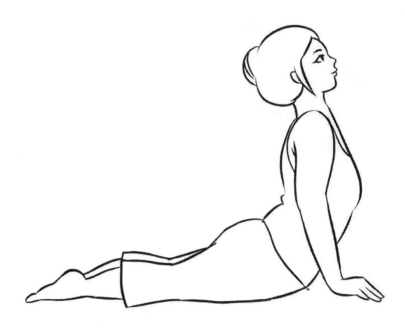

As a child, I often used to adopt a variation of this pose to get comfortable whilst reading a book. We spend so much time bending forwards, that backward bends of any kind are really beneficial for our lower backs, muscles in the chest, shoulders and tummy, and also our bottoms. Best of all, it makes us feel great and can alleviate any menstrual pain we might be suffering from.

1. From the Low Plank position, lower your knees to the floor, flip your feet over, followed by your chest and push upwards with the crown of your head.

2. Point your toes and imagine your body extending from the tips of your toes to the crown of your head.

3. Check in with your body, making sure your hands are directly under your shoulders, and your shoulder-blades are pulled down and away from your ears.

4. Inhale, lifting your chest up and tightening your stomach and thigh muscles to help you feel strong and supple. Then exhale.

5. Hold for 2-3 whole breaths.

6. There are several modifications you can make in this pose. If your thighs get in the way feel free to move your legs apart slightly. If your wrists tire, try popping a blanket underneath your hands or even resting down onto your forearms instead. Feel free to experiment a little and find what feels best for you.

Downward Facing Dog

Adho Mukha Svanasana

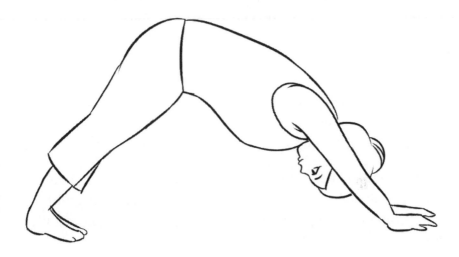

Downward Facing Dog is one of the classic yoga poses that I absolutely adore. It ticks all of the usual boxes - being amazing for your back, strength and balance. But it's also brilliant for your hamstrings, helps minimize headache and migraine attacks, calms and centers your body, and just feels good!

My friends often struggle with 'the boob problem' when practicing this asana. Boobs can be fond of heading towards your face and attempting to suffocate you. Instead, invest in a sturdy sports bra or two, or even consider using a belt or strap wrapped across your body and under your arms. This will do the trick - I promise.

1. From Cobra Pose, push yourself back onto your hands and knees and flip your feet over so your toes are tucked underneath.

2. Walk your hands a few inches forward and spread your fingers as wide as you can and ground into the floor.

3. On your next exhale, lift your knees from the floor, push your tailbone high towards to ceiling, and try to ground down through your feet (although don't expect them to touch the floor immediately). Your body should form a 'V' shape.

4. Check in with your body, pressing your shoulders away from your ears, keeping your feet hip-width apart and your knees slightly bent. Feel your body lift and lengthen.

5. Hold for 3 whole breaths.

6. For sore wrists and hands, try playing a block under each hand, resting on a folded towel, or even resting on your elbows instead of your hands.

7. Tight hamstrings? Don't get too hung-up on getting your legs to stay straight and making those feet touch the ground. If anything hurts, or you feel too tight, bend those knees a little.

Low Lunge
Anjaneyasana

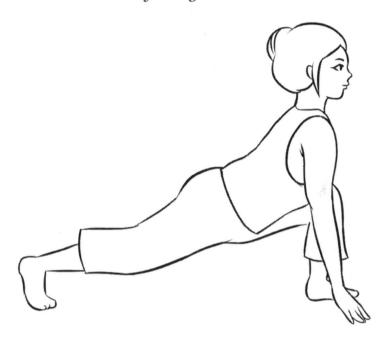

We're on the home-stretch now, returning to where we started at the beginning of the sequence. Again, for back problems, sciatica and the general aches and pains that can pop up - this posture is wonderful. Sink into it to feel a deep stretch through your hips, groin and legs. You're getting there!

1. From Downward Facing Dog, lift your head and look forwards between your hands. Exhale and step forwards with your left foot, bending at the knee. Check your alignment here and make sure that your foot is directly under your knee. Depending on your body shape and flexibility, you might not be able to smoothly move that leg forwards. Instead, consider taking it forwards in lots of small steps, lower your right knee to the floor to provide you with extra support, or even take that foot out wide as you move it forwards.

2. Grab those blocks again and place them by your sides (if needed), and press through your hands, opening your fingers wide to help you to balance.

3. Move your shoulders away from your ears, engage your stomach muscles and look forwards ahead of you.

4. Hold the pose for 5 breaths.

Standing Forward Bend

Uttanasana

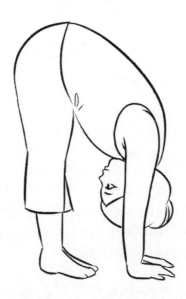

As mentioned the first time around, this might well be my favorite asana of them all. Again, it looks mighty simple but it can be quite challenging and highly beneficial for your entire body. It's the perfect way to de-stress and help overcome mild depression. As well as stretching those hamstrings and calves, it will also do wonders for any symptoms of the menopause, high blood pressure, infertility or headaches and migraines.

1. From Low Lunge, bring your right foot to join your left, keeping your hands on the floor or on those blocks as best you can.

2. Now exhale and imagine yourself folding forward from your hip joints, lengthening through the crown of your head and extending down toward your feet.

3. If your belly gets in the way at this point, use your hands to tuck it gently out of the way, widen your legs, and try again. Widen your legs if you need to, but make sure your feet stay parallel.

4. Again, don't get too hung up on touching those toes - that will come in time. Draw in your tummy muscles, and lengthen that torso towards the ground.

5. We will be moving towards getting those legs straight, but for now, bend them as deeply as you need to in order to support the rest of your body.

6. For additional arm support, bring in a pair of blocks and place your hands upon them.

7. Relax your head and neck and allow your head to hand loosely towards the ground. Don't forget to breathe.

8. Hold this pose for 5 breaths, depending on how comfortable you feel.

Upward Salute

Urdhva Hastasana

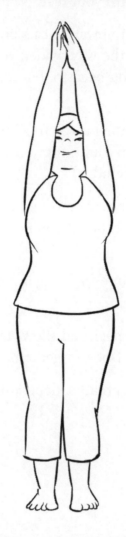

We arrive back to the pose that provides the perfect warm-up stretch for your entire body. It's great for asthma, back ache and fatigue as it helps open up the lungs, extend and nourish the spine and get everything moving as it should in the digestive system.

1. From Standing Forward Bend, engage your stomach muscles and begin to peel yourself up vertebra - by-vertebra until you have reached a standing position. Keep your shoulders relaxed and away from your ears, and keep grounding down through your feet.

2. Take a deep breath and raise your hands overhead, palms still touching. Reach towards the sky. Don't worry if you're tighter in the shoulders and your hands won't touch - just keep them parallel and reach as high as you can.

3. Without compressing your neck, tip your head back slightly and gaze upwards. If you find your balance suffers, return to looking directly ahead of you, close your eyes and breathe.

4. Hold for five breaths before moving into the next posture.

Mountain Pose

Tadasana

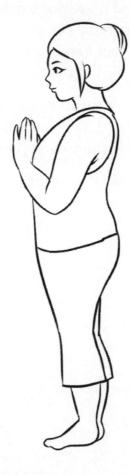

And now we're right back to where we started! You should be very proud of yourself, and hopefully excited about what yoga can offer you. Let's round things up.

1. To conclude, draw your hands down from above you and hold them just in front of your chest, thumbs touching your breastbone.

2. Keep your feet firmly on the ground, shoulders pulled back down from your ears and crown of your head gently pulled towards the sky.

3. Pay attention to your feet and either move them together until they are touching from your big toe right back to your heel, or otherwise placed hip width apart. Make sure they are parallel and facing forward.

4. Take a deep breath and allow the air fill up your lungs from the very bottom, into your belly, into your chest and right up under your shoulders. Then exhale slowly.

5. Stay in the pose for a further four breaths.

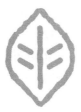

QUICK RECAP

- Sun salutations are a flow of several yoga postures, or *asanas,* which work together to awaken the body, encourage flexibility, muscle strength and calm and sooth the nervous system.

- Move through each of the postures outlined in this section one by one, paying close attention to your body alignment and taking your unique body needs into consideration.

- Once you have finished one round of sun salutations, ideally you need to repeat the sequence on the other side. To be a true yogi, you should also aim to complete at least 2 to 4 rounds per day on both sides.

- Don't be afraid to modify any of the postures in the ways suggested, using blocks, rolled up blankets, small cushions, or physically moving any skin or wobbly bits out of the way with your hands.

- Never feel that you have replicate the images provided. These are meant to be only a guide for you, so that you understand the final body shape we are aiming for. Everyone has their own best version of a pose, so your aim should be to work towards this instead of some photographic ideal.

- ***NEED A REST?*** Yoga might look easy, but it's a lot of hard work. So don't feel discouraged if you get tired during your practice. Simply rest back into Child's Pose, or find someplace to rest before you restart your practice.

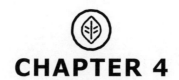

CHAPTER 4

Troubleshooting:
Yoga For Winter Blues & Depression

The following five postures are all you need to shake off the winter blues, get your blood flowing and help to shift you from a place of internal darkness, to positivity and sunshine.

In themselves they form an excellent short practice that you can use on its own when you aren't feeling your best. You can also add them to a sun salutation routine, but keep in mind than many of these postures are already included in the sun salutation.

If you really are struggling with low mood, aim to get moving as much as possible and get outside in the sunlight at least once per day if you can. It will make a huge difference to how you are feeling.

Upward Salute

Urdhva Hastasana

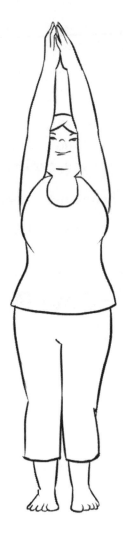

You have already seen this posture in the previous section on Sun Salutations, and now you will use it to beat your winter blues. It's so effective because it opens up your entire body, allows for circulation to flow freely and feels like an awakening for your entire body.

1. Stand on your mat with your feet together, touching from big toe to heel. If this is difficult, you can take them slightly apart. Adjust to feel comfortable. Make sure your shoulders are relaxed and away from your ears, and keep grounding down through your feet.

2. Take a deep breath and raise your hands overhead, palms still touching. Reach towards the sky. Don't worry if you're a little tight in the shoulders and your hands won't touch - just keep them parallel and reach as high as you can.

3. Without compressing your neck, tip your head back slightly and gaze upwards. If you find your balance suffers, return to looking directly ahead of you, close your eyes and breathe.

4. Hold for five breaths before moving into the next posture.

Cat-Cow Pose

Chakravakasana

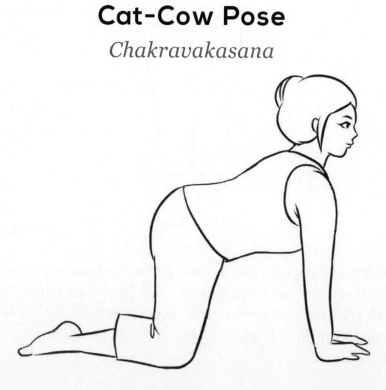

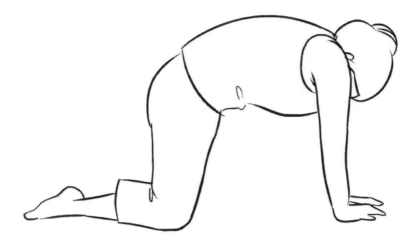

Cat-Cow is a classic yoga pose which gently guides your spine through its full range of movement and helps release trapped tension, tackles back-pain, gets your circulation moving and also calms and focuses your body and mind. Let's take a look at how we can do it.

1. Get onto your hands and knees and make yourself comfortable. If your knees are feeling sore, roll up a small blanket and place it underneath for extra support.

2. Make sure your hands are directly beneath your shoulders and your knees are directly beneath your hips. Keep your back long and make sure those shoulders aren't creeping up towards your ears.

3. Take a deep breath, and as you do so, lift your bottom to the sky and allow your belly to drop towards the floor. Look up towards the sky and picture your spine forming an imaginary 'U' shape.

4. As you exhale, round your spine and feel an imaginary string pull it towards to sky. Tuck your head down, towards your belly button and allow your hands and the tops of your feet to push you up from the ground.

5. On the next inhale repeat the entire sequence; allowing your belly to drop on the inhale and arch towards the sky on the exhale.

6. Repeat a total of 5 whole breaths.

Downward Facing Dog
Adho Mukha Svanasana

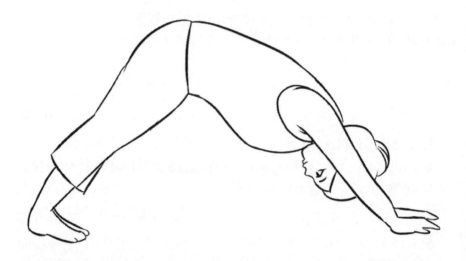

Again we revisit the Downward Facing Dog, which is one of the classic yoga poses that I absolutely adore. It ticks all of the usual boxes - being amazing for your back, strength and balance. Most importantly for you now, it calms and centers your entire body, and just feels good!

As mentioned in the Sun Salutations chapter, many of my friends often struggle with 'the boob problem' when practicing this asana. Boobs can be fond of heading towards your face and attempting to suffocate you. Instead, invest in a sturdy sports bra or two, or even consider using a belt or strap wrapped across your body and under your arms.

1. From Cat-Cow Pose, walk your hands a few inches forward and spread your fingers as wide as you can and ground into the floor.

2. On your next exhale, lift your knees from the floor, push your tailbone high towards to ceiling, and try to ground down through your feet (although don't expect them to touch the floor immediately). Your body should form a 'V' shape.

3. Check in with your body, pressing your shoulders away from your ears, keeping your feet hip-width apart and your knees slightly bent. Feel your body lift and lengthen.

4. Hold for 5 whole breaths.

5. For sore wrists and hands, try playing a block under each hand, resting on a folded towel, or even resting on your elbows instead of your hands.

6. Tight hamstrings? Don't get too hung-up on getting your legs to stay straight and making those feet touch the ground. If anything hurts, or you feel too tight, bend those knees a little.

Legs-Up-The-Wall Pose
Viparita Karani

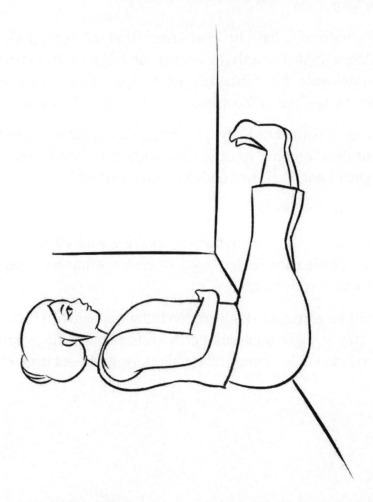

When you've been on your feet all day, or are feeling stressed and even a little overwhelmed with life, move into this posture. It's fantastic for relieving tired or cramped legs, stretches out those hamstrings and provides you an opportunity to disconnect and relax - no questions asked. If you only do one yoga pose for your stress, depression and anxiety, make it this one!

1. Sit beside a wall, with your right side touching that wall. Breathe out and swing your legs up and around until they are resting on the wall.

2. Shuffle your bottom as close to the wall as you can, and rest back into the pose.

3. Ideally, you need to hold this pose for 5 to 10 minutes but less time will also be effective.

4. To modify the pose, grab a pillow or blanket, fold it up and pop it beneath your bottom. You can also move slightly away from the wall if your hamstrings are particularly tight. Place a small pillow beneath your head if you feel more comfortable.

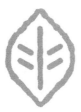

Child's Pose
Balasana

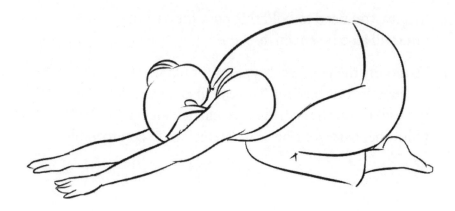

Child's Pose is the most restorative pose of them all, and is one you will grow to love. As your yoga practice becomes more challenging and you feel stretched beyond your comfort zone, Child's Pose is the place you will return to. It's relaxing, calming, and brilliant for keeping your back healthy.

1. Settle yourself down onto the floor and get into a kneeling position. If your ankle or knees complain loudly, pop a folded-up blanket or small pillow under your bottom. If this doesn't do the trick, instead keep those feet close together but take your knees out wide to the side.

2. Now pop your arms in front of you, hands touching the ground.

3. Lean your body forward and down towards the ground as much as you can. Resist the urge to force yourself forward - just allow yourself to melt forward, releasing all tension from your body. Let your tummy rest either on your thigh, or between them, depending on which variation you are going for.

4. If you're already flexible, allow your forehead to rest on the floor. Pop a blanket underneath if this feels uncomfortable, and continue to let your body melt into the floor.

5. You can hold this pose for as long as you need. Why not try 5 breaths, or extend if you feel good in the pose?

I hope you've enjoyed this troubleshooting chapter dedicated to blowing the cobwebs away, uplifting your spirits and helping to shift any mild depression and/or anxiety that might be lurking inside. Next we turn our attention to that all-important subject of sleep - which poses can help improve your nightly slumber? Find out in the next chapter.

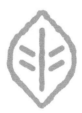

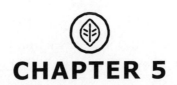

CHAPTER 5

Troubleshooting:
Yoga For Better Sleep

Sleep is one of the absolute essentials in life - without it you just won't function or feel like yourself. So if you are having trouble getting to sleep, staying asleep or waking early in the morning, yoga might just be the solution you are looking for.

It works by resting and relaxing your body and mind, helps to rebalance your sleep hormones and benefits your brain and nervous system as a whole. Research conducted at *Harvard Medical School, Boston*, offers proof that yoga really is effective at treating insomnia and inducing relaxation.

Again, use the following poses as an add-on to a sun salutation practice, or enjoy them as part of your bedtime routine to help you unwind from your day, only to wake the next morning feeling refreshed and raring to go.

Easy Pose With Forward Bend

Adho Mukha Sukhasana

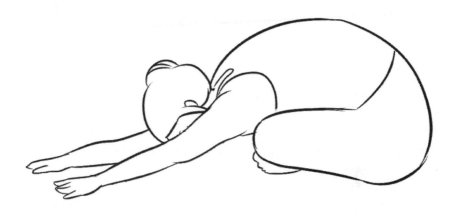

This posture is perfect for releasing tension from your entire body, as well as reducing anxiety and fatigue and helping you to disconnect from your day. Practice this and you will feel physically and mentally ready for some blissful shut-eye.

1. Sit on the floor and cross your legs beneath you. It doesn't matter which leg goes on top, just as long as you are comfortable. If you find it difficult at this stage to fold your legs, use your fingers to push the skin behind your knees gently out of the way, and then try again. You can also choose to sit in a straight-backed chair instead, with your feet flat on the ground and back held straight.

2. Pay attention to the position of your bottom on the floor (or chair). Ground your entire body by rooting through your sit-bones and feel yourself being pulled high towards the sky, as if you have a string attached to the crown of your head. Adjust your buttocks if they prevent your sit-bones from touching the floor.

3. Now lift those shoulders back and down, away from your ears, and gently lift your breastbone towards the sky.

4. Inhale. Then as you exhale start to walk your hands out in front of you as far as you can, keeping your sit bones on the floor. Release your head and neck to relax completely.

5. Hold for 5 breaths, then repeat with your legs crossed in the opposite direction.

6. Straighten out the legs and repeat with the left shin in front, followed by the right shin.

7. If you find your sit bones lifting, consider supporting them with a small pillow, a rolled-up blanket or even blocks.

Plow Pose (With Chair)

Halasana

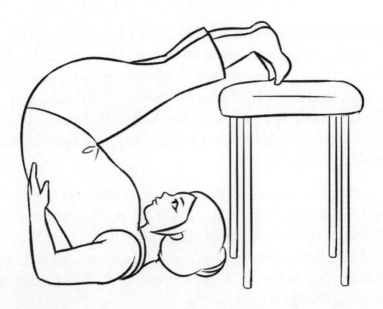

This is a modification of the classic Plow Pose, which asks you to place your feet on the floor behind your head. However, getting feet so far over can be challenging for a beginner, especially if you are on the curvier side. But of course, we still want to enjoy the benefits and this modification will help you do just that. It relaxes your brain and nervous system, stimulates your digestions, stretches your spine, reduces stress and helps you to fall asleep more easily. Let's find out how.

1. Grab a chair and place it at the top of your mat above the place you intend your head to be when you lie down.

2. Lie on the mat with your head facing towards the chair, your arms beside you.

3. Inhale, then use your tummy muscles to pull your legs into the air, high above you. Allow your legs to swing over your head and rest lightly on the chair behind you.

4. Soften your throat and try to extend your neck as much as possible. Use your hands to support your hips and rest your elbows on the floor beneath you.

5. Hold this pose for five breaths.

6. To exit this pose, move your hands back to the floor and swing your legs back over your head and to the floor.

Standing Forward Bend

Uttanasana

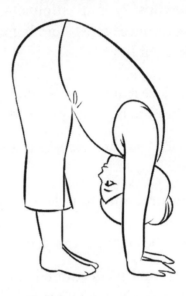

As mentioned the first time around, this pose might seem simple but it can be quite challenging - yet highly beneficial for your entire body. It's the perfect way to de-stress and help overcome mild depression. As well as stretching those hamstrings and calves, it will also do wonders for any symptoms of the menopause, high blood pressure, infertility or headaches and migraines.

1. Bring your right foot to join your left, keeping your hands on the floor or on those blocks as best you can.

2. Now exhale and imagine yourself folding forward from your hip joints, lengthening through the crown of your head and extending down toward your feet.

3. If your belly gets in the way at this point, use your hands to tuck it gently out of the way, widen your legs, and try again.

Widen your legs if you need to, but make sure your feet stay parallel.

4. Again, don't get too hung up on touching those toes - that will come in time. Draw in your tummy muscles, and lengthen that torso towards the ground.

5. We will be moving towards getting those legs straight, but for now, bend them as deeply as you need to in order to support the rest of your body.

6. For additional arm support, bring in a pair of blocks and place your hands upon them.

7. Relax your head and neck and allow your head to hang loosely towards the ground. Don't forget to breathe.

8. Hold this pose for 5 breaths, depending on how comfortable you feel.

Supine Spinal Twist

Supta Matsyendrasana

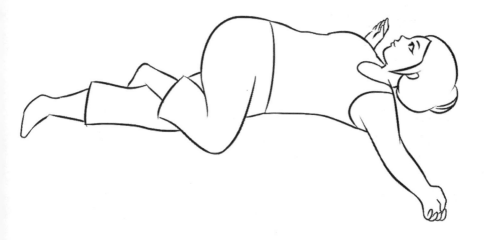

No matter how relaxed and loose I *think* my back is, I can guarantee that this pose will result in a satisfying (and pain-free) 'click' - which releases a ton of tension and helps me feel brand-new. I'm sure you're going to love it too. It benefits your back, eases tightness in your shoulders, improves your digestion and also calms and quietens your mind, helping you enjoy a brilliant night's sleep.

1. Gently position yourself to lie down on the floor or on your mat.

2. Bend your knees and place the soles of your feet on the floor. Then lift your right knee up towards your chest, keeping that left leg planted firmly on the ground.

3. Turn your attention to that right knee again and drop it over to the left side of your body, aiming to move it towards the floor whilst keeping that left shoulder down on the ground too.

4. Open your arms wide beside you and allow your body to relax into the posture. You might find that your knee doesn't want to touch the floor, and that is perfectly fine. Simply slip a small cushion or two under that knee to offer some support.

5. Stay in this posture for 5 breaths.

Corpse Pose

Savasana

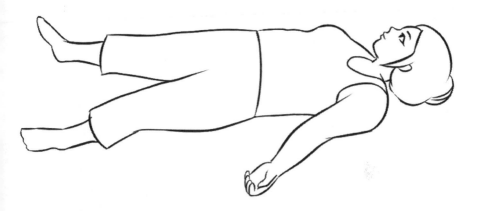

This pose might look easy, but it can often be the most challenging of the asanas. Relaxing isn't often as easy as flicking a switch and many people struggle to settle. Relaxation is truly an art, and Corpse Pose will help you develop this gift. It will also help relieve stress and mild depression, reduce headaches and migraines and helps to lower blood pressure. Here's how.

1. Grab a blanket and lie on your mat, legs a comfortable distance apart and arms resting loosely by your sides. Place that blanket under your head or use it as a cover whilst you relax.

2. Allow your feet and hands to fall sideways and open up. Close your eyes and take several deep breaths.

3. Turn your attention to the muscles throughout your body. Start by noticing your face and relaxing each of your muscles in turn, then you neck, your torso, your arms, your legs, your groin; every single one of your muscles. Also pay attention to your tongue your nostrils, the bridge of your nose and your ears.

4. Allow your eyes to rest back and allow your mind to rest.

5. Stay in this pose for at least 5 minutes, if not more.

6. Don't be surprised if you mind tries to wander - it will probably try to fight against the silence and persuade you to get up and move, or think about what to buy at the supermarket tomorrow. Don't let it. This is your time to relax, to move towards the sleep you deserve.

The postures we have covered in this section are practically guaranteed to help you achieve that blissful, rejuvenating sleep that you deserve. Go on and try one out tonight - you'll be amazed at the results.

Our next chapter turns its attention to the ever-popular topic of weight loss. Even if you're very happy with your body, it's really worth practicing all of the postures. By doing this, you'll expand your own yoga knowledge and increase your flexibility as well as benefit your mental and physical health in so many ways.

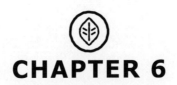

CHAPTER 6

Troubleshooting:
Yoga For Weight Loss

You might be surprised to hear that yoga is great for weight loss too. Whilst it's true to say that it burns around 3-6 calories per minute, it also boasts more amazing benefits. These include greater body awareness, an increased level of mindfulness, stronger muscles (which in turn helps burn more fat), better strength and self-esteem and also that all-important one, stress management. You will feel more centered as a person and empowered to make the right food and lifestyle choices for your body, finally breaking free of any emotional eating patterns. Let's take a look.

Cobbler Pose

Badhakonasana

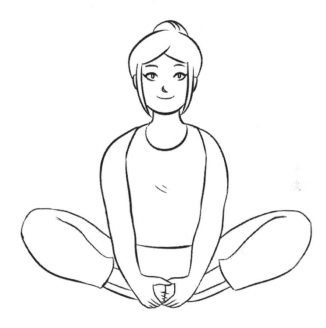

This asana helps tone your inner thighs and strengthens your spine, muscles of the groin, knees and lower back. It also helps relieve menstrual discomfort and improves digestion.

1. Sit on the floor or on your mat with your legs stretched out in front of you. Keep that spine nice and tall.

2. Now bend your legs at the knees, being sure to tuck any skin out of the way using your fingers so that you can be more comfortable.

3. Move your feet together and allow your soles close together in front of you. If this feels uncomfortable, move your feet slightly away from you and try again.

4. Hold onto your feet and gently move your knees up and down slightly to allow you to gain more space in those muscles.

5. Repeat as many times as comfortably can.

6. Pop a blanket or pillow under your bottom if you are feeling uncomfortable or finding it tricky to sit up straight.

Sage Pose

Vasishtasana

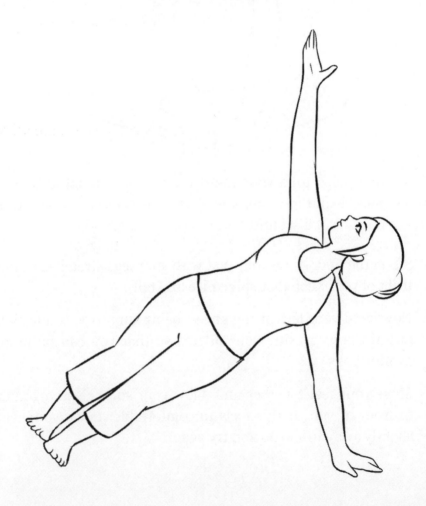

Sage Pose looks amazing once you master it, but it does take some strength and focus to accomplish. I promise you that any effort you invest will pay off well. This pose will help trim down your waistline, tone your muscles in your stomach, strengthen your shoulders and arms and help you feel athletic and powerful. Here's how to do it.

1. Lie down on your stomach on the floor.

2. Bend your elbows, make sure your palms are beneath your shoulders, tuck your toes under and push yourself up into a Plank Pose.

3. Now release your left hand from the floor and twist your upper body around to the left. Lift your hand high towards the sky and look up towards it.

4. At the same time, turn your right foot onto its side and allow your left foot to rest on top of it.

5. Stay in this position for five breaths, then repeat on the other side.

Half Moon Pose

Ardha Chandrasana

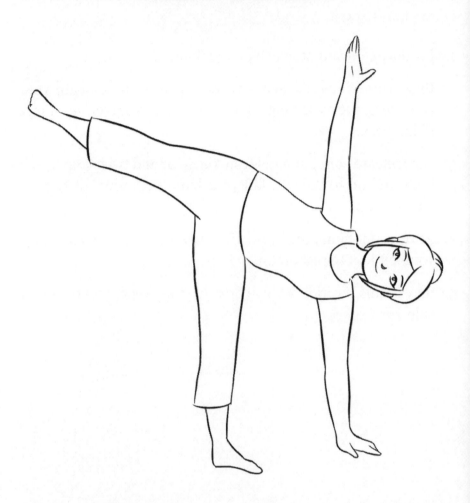

This pose is great to tone your buttocks, upper and inner thighs, and mastering it will give you an incredible sense of achievement. It helps target lower back pain, strengthens your back, legs, hips, and abdomen, and also eases PMT. Plus you really will feel like a bendy pretzel! Give it a go.

1. Stand on your mat and place your feet together.

2. Step your left foot back several inches, and as you do this, place your right hand on the floor, slightly ahead of your right food. Use a block if this is tricky to achieve.

3. Exhale and as you do so, lift that left leg up high, engaging all of the muscles in your leg and reaching backwards through its length.

4. Pop your left hand on your hip for added stability, or if you are feeling brave, extend that hand above you, reaching towards the sky.

5. Hold for around 3 breaths then repeat on the other side.

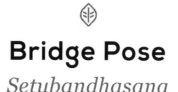

Bridge Pose
Setubandhasana

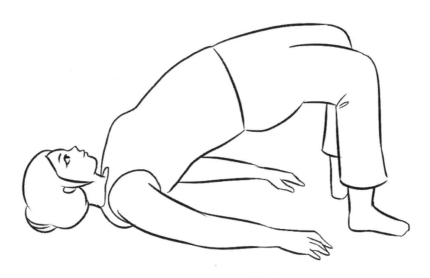

Bridge Pose is so amazing for weight-loss because it is beneficial so many parts of your body, as well as your mind. Not only does it extend your spine and stretches your chest and thighs, but it also boosts your digestion, helps lower your blood pressure, and releases an enormous amount of tension that can often trigger comfort eating and other issues with food. Here's how to do it.

1. Lie down on the floor with your knees bent directly over your heels for added alignment.

2. Rest your arms down on the ground at your sides, palms down and shoulders relaxed away from your ears.

3. Exhale then lift your hips and thighs high into the air. You aim is to get them as high as you can, but as you have probably guessed, this is much harder than it looks. For added support underneath your bottom, place a folded blanket or a small pillow beneath you.

4. Hold this position for 5 breaths.

Warrior I

Virabhadrasana I

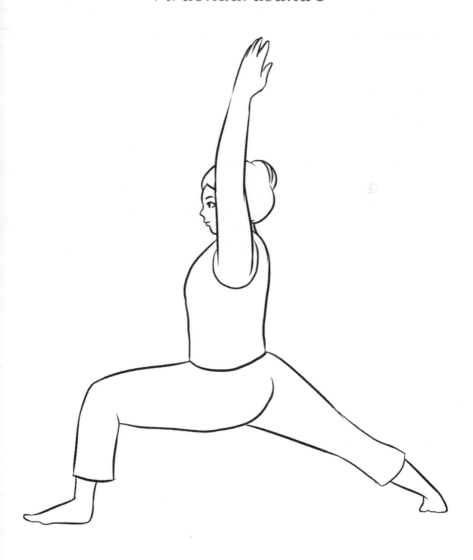

This is one of a collection of three poses that help you to unleash your inner power. In this section we will just concentrate on one: the aptly-named Warrior I. It might not look like much, but it has a powerful effect upon your body and mind. It's an effective way to stretch your legs, groins, shoulders and neck and strengthens them at the same time. This pose will help you feel empowered and ready to take on the world.

1. Stand with your legs around one meter apart (3-4 feet) and turn your right foot out to 90 degrees and your left foot in slightly.

2. Rest your hands down on your hips, relax those shoulders away from your ears.

3. Check in with your posture and make sure that your knee is directly over your hip, your hips are facing directly forwards and draw your tailbone down and towards the floor.

4. If you're feeling off balance and a bit wobbly, practice the asana next to a wall and hold on when you need to!

5. If you are feeling brave, sweep your hands up and over your head, meeting in the middle with palms touching.

6. Hold for 5 breaths before switching to the other side.

Tree Pose

Vrksasana

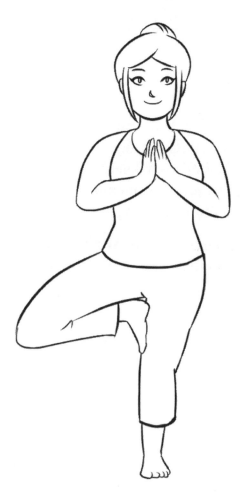

This posture is harder than it looks, but it works wonders for your entire body and mind. Firstly, it helps to strengthen all of those muscles in your thighs, calves and spine which will help you feel stronger and shift those excess pounds. Secondly, it boosts your power of focus, improves your quality of sleep and helps to calm and relax your mind. Lastly, it relieves any trapped muscles or nerves, relieving sciatica and releasing tension in the spine and shoulders. You'll feel like a goddess when you practice this one. Here's how to do it.

1. From Warrior I, lower your arms to your sides and step your back foot up to meet the front one and center yourself.

2. Now shift your weight onto your left foot and ground down through all four 'corners' of your feet, feeling strong and stable.

3. Bend your right leg and reach down to grab your ankle. Tuck any skin out of the way with your fingers, and get comfortable.

4. Using your hands, lift up your leg and place your right foot directly onto your thigh, as high as you feel comfortable. Avoid resting your foot on your knee, and instead place it slightly higher or slightly lower. Remember, this is not a competition. No one is watching or keeping score.

5. Remove your hands and either place them together in front of you, on your hips, or rest on a wall beside you to help you maintain your balance.

6. Lengthen your spine and draw your tailbone down towards the floor, fixing your eyes on one point directly ahead of you. This will help you keep your balance.

7. Hold for 5 breaths, and then repeat on the other side.

8. Don't feel discouraged if you wobble around and can barely lift your foot from the ground at first. This is perfectly normal and you will progress over time - I promise. For now, use the wall or the back of a chair to help.

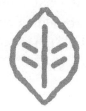

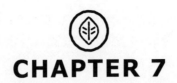

CHAPTER 7

Troubleshooting:
Yoga For Period Pain

When it's that 'time of the month', it can be hard to concentrate on anything except the gripping, aching feeling low in your tummy. This short series of yoga postures will help you ease that period pain without resorting to painkillers or just trying to put up with it. Best of all, they all help you feel relaxed, calm and rebalanced at this point in your cycle. I've personally suffered with period pain most of my life, and it wasn't until I cleaned up my diet, experimented with herbal remedies and discovered yoga that I was able to effectively tackle it. I'm sure you'll enjoy the same brilliant benefits. Let's take a look.

Head-To-Knee Forward Bend
Janu Sirsasana A

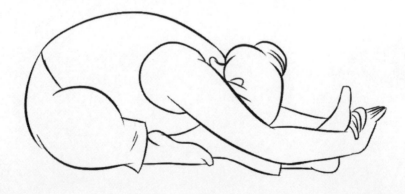

Allow yourself to melt forward into this pose to ease your period pain, relieve symptoms of menopause, calm your mind, reduce anxiety and help you get a better night's sleep. This pose is utterly relaxing, as well as effective at targeting those hamstrings and bottom. Here's how to do it.

1. Sit yourself down on the floor and extend those legs straight out in front of you.

2. Bend your left knee, tucking away any excess skin that might get in the way, and place the sole of your left foot close to your right inner thigh.

3. Check in with your posture - make sure you are lengthening up through your spine, your hips are square and those shoulders are down away from your ears.

4. As you exhale, fold forwards from the hips and extend up and over your extended leg. Avoid the temptation to get your head to touch your leg - that will come in time. Concentrate on elongating the spine.

5. If you can, reach forwards towards your toes, grasp them and gently pull them towards you, whilst grounding through your left heel.

6. Stay in this pose for 5 breaths before repeating on the other side.

Camel Pose

Ustrasana

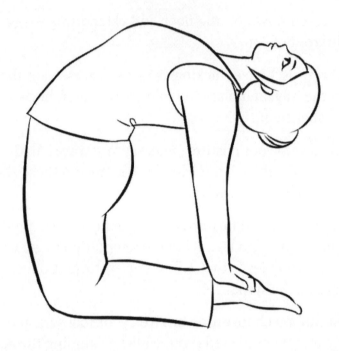

For an intense energy boost and relief from your menstrual aches and pains, give this amazing posture a try. It helps release and nourish your inner organs (including your female organs), stretches out that chest and helps your spine become more flexible. It's not the easiest of poses to achieve, but don't let that put you off. You can still enjoy it and ease your discomfort.

1. Kneel down on the floor and move your knees so that they are hip-width apart. Pop a blanket or a pillow beneath your knees if you are feeling sore.

2. Press your legs into the floor to help you with balance, and rest your hands onto the back of your hips and breathe.

3. Then take a deep breath, lift up that chest and press your shoulders down.

4. As you exhale, push your hips forward and reach back with your hands towards your heels. The final aim will be to actually touch your heels, but don't expect this to happen overnight. Use blocks to give you that extra support should you need it.

5. Stabilize your position, pressing your legs down towards the floor. Rest your hands on the back of your hips (place the base of your palms on the top part of your glutes and point your fingers down). Inhale, lift your chest, and press your shoulders down, towards the ribs.

6. Drop your head back and continue to breathe deeply and calmly.

7. Stay in this position for 5 breaths and come out very gently, vertebra-by-vertebra.

Reclining Bound-Angle Pose

Supta Baddha Konasana

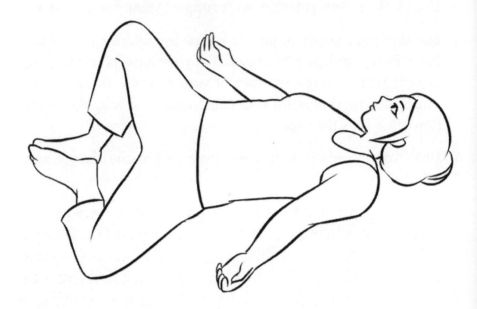

This pose is relaxing and calming yet stimulates your internal abdominal organs, your ovaries, bladder and kidneys, and is an effective way to stop your suffering. It will also give your inner thighs and knees a wonderful stretch and help boost your circulation, so you feel more grounded and alive. As you might have noticed, it's very similar to Cobbler Pose, but reclining this time instead. Here's how to do it.

1. Start by sitting yourself gently down on the floor, on top of a mat or other soft surface.

2. Stretch your legs out in front of you, keep that spine nice and tall and rooting down through your sit bones. Pop a cushion, rolled up mat or small pillow under your bottom if needed.

3. Now bend your legs at the knees, being sure to tuck any skin out of the way using your fingers so that you can be more comfortable.

4. Move your feet together and press your soles close together in front of you. If this feels uncomfortable, move your feet away slightly and try again.

5. Now here comes the new bit. Exhale and lower your back towards the floor very slowly. Ease yourself into it bit by bit and make sure you aren't pushing yourself too hard. If you can't yet make it all the way to the floor, stay resting on your hands or elbows for now, or rest your head on a pillow instead to help.

6. Use your hands and touch the top of your thighs, rotating them slightly towards the middle.

7. Push your knees sideways away from your knees, and imagine your groin melting towards the ground. If you feel a great strain in that inner thigh area, consider raising your feet with a block.

8. When you are happy and in your best version of the pose, relax and breathe.

9. Stay in the pose for 5 breaths, increasing the number of breaths as you become more flexible.

Half Lord-Of-The-Fishes Pose
Ardha Matsyendrasana

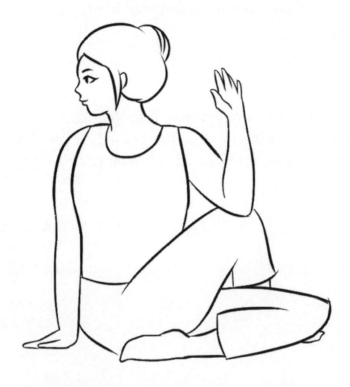

Period pain teamed with a busy life can leave your entire body feeling out-of-sorts and in need of some TLC. This wonderful stretching pose will help you reclaim your body and your muscles, energize your spine and simulate your internal organs, like your womb, your liver and your kidneys. This posture is perfect for bedtime as it also ensures deep and restful sleep. Give it a try!

1. Settle down on the floor and extend those legs out in front of you. Support your bottom with a small cushion or folded up blanket.

2. Bend your right leg, bringing it up close to your bottom. Notice how your left leg is still extended in front of you.

3. Now shift your weight slightly onto your left leg and bring it under your bent knee and around towards your right buttocks. It can be helpful to refer to the illustration if you need to.

4. Make sure that right foot is firmly pressed into the floor, your right knee is pointing up towards to the sky, and your left leg is next to your hip.

5. Inhale and feel yourself growing taller towards to sky, spine extending upwards and space growing between your vertebra.

6. Now exhale and twist your body around towards your right thigh. Place your right hand on the floor to help you gain extra stability. Bend your left arm, tucking it on the outside side of your right thigh. Don't force or pull anything, just settle into this position.

7. Check in with your body - press that right foot into the floor, release your groin, get those shoulders away from your ears and allow your head to follow the direction of the twist.

8. Hold for 5 breaths, allowing each inhale to help you extend your spine upwards and giving you that extra space to twist.

As you have seen in this chapter, you absolutely don't have to suffer with period pain without being able to do anything about it. Yoga is a powerful way to target any menstrual problems you might be having, whether it's period pain, PMT, or even infertility. Make sure you include these asanas in your monthly practice, and you will feel so much better.

We're nearing the end of the book, but there is just time to squeeze in a quick sequence that you can do to fix your mood, energize your body, and generally de-stress whenever you need to. All it takes is 5 minutes and you'll soon be feeling much better. Turn to the next chapter to find out how.

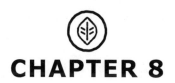

CHAPTER 8

Troubleshooting:
Gentle 5-Minute-Fix Yoga

Have you ever checked the clock and realized that you've spent almost the entire day hunched over your computer screen and as a result, your back and head are both screaming *"STOP! For goodness sake!"* in desperation? Or perhaps your body is out-of-sorts and needs a good dose of TLC and a massage? Or maybe you've sat in front of a great movie or two and need to get yourself up and moving? If so, this short section will be absolutely perfect for you.

The following four *asanas* are wonderfully gentle and restorative, yet effective enough to get that blood flowing and ease your aches and pains. It's a fab 5-minute fix that you can do (almost) anywhere. Let's take a look.

Easy Pose

Sukhasana

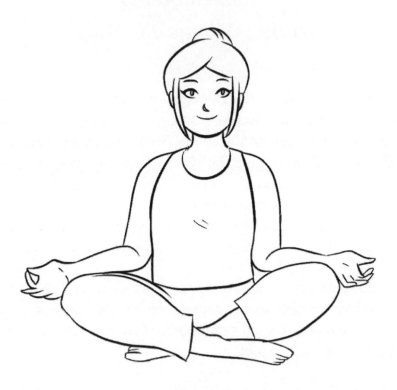

This pose will help you disconnect from the stresses, strains and obligations of everyday life for a few moments and help you press the 'reset' button on whatever you are doing. It helps you to become more focused, grounded, and also promotes excellent posture and calmness.

1. Sit on the floor and cross your legs beneath you. It doesn't matter which leg goes on top, just as long as you are comfortable. If you find it difficult at the moment to fold your legs, use your fingers to push the skin behind your knees gently out of the way, and then try again. You can also choose to sit

in a straight-backed chair instead, with your feet flat on the ground and back held straight.

2. Now rest your hands gently on your knees, with your palms facing upwards.

3. Pay attention to the position of your bottom on the floor (or chair). Ground your entire body by rooting through your sit-bones and feel yourself being pulled high towards the sky, as if you have a string attached to the crown of your head. Adjust your buttocks if they prevent your sit-bones from touching the floor or grab a cushion or folded-up blanket if they feel sore.

4. Now lift those shoulders back and down, away from your ears, and gently lift your breastbone towards the sky.

5. Check in with your entire body - pull your shoulders down from your ears, mentally check all of your muscles for any sign of tension and relax each of them in turn.

6. Hold the pose for five breaths.

Seated Twist

Parivrtta sukhasana

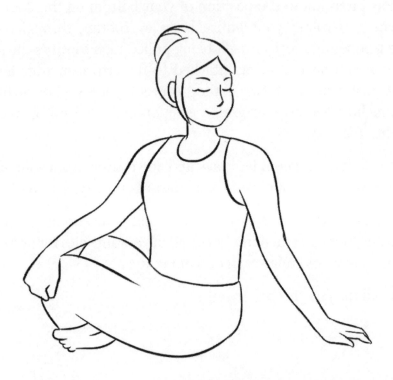

This asana will increase the circulation throughout your body, nourish your spine and keep it flexible, and also help strengthen and streamline your tummy muscles. It's my own favorite pose for those computer days, or even when I've spent a bunch of time traveling.

1. Sit on the floor with your legs extended.

2. Now cross your legs, again, get comfortable and feel free to move any skin out of the way, using your fingers. You can also choose to sit in a straight-backed chair instead, with your feet flat on the ground and back held straight.

3. Place your left hand on the ground next to you, a small distance away from your body and place your right hand on your right knee.

4. Root those sit-bone down onto the ground and lift yourself tall through that imaginary string in the top of your head. Keeping that height, twist your body around to the left, keeping both buttocks firmly on the floor. Allow your head to move towards the same direction as your shoulders.

5. Stay in this position for around one minute, or less if uncomfortable for you.

6. Repeat on the other side.

Cat-Cow Pose

Chakravakasana

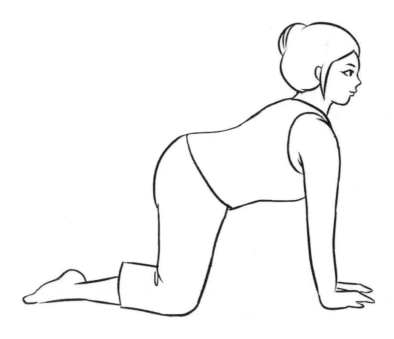

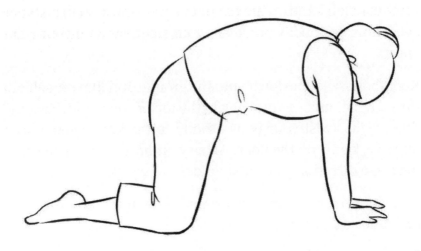

As we touched on earlier on, Cat-Cow Pose is a classic yoga pose which gently guides your spine through its full range of movement and helps release trapped tension, tackles back-pain, gets your circulation moving and also calms and focuses your body and mind.

1. Get onto your hands and knees and make yourself comfortable. If your knees are feeling sore, roll up a small blanket and place it underneath for extra support.

2. Make sure your hands are directly beneath your shoulders and your knees are directly beneath your hips. Keep your back long and make sure those shoulders aren't creeping up towards your ears.

3. Take a deep breath, and as you do so, lift your bottom to the sky and allow your belly to drop towards the floor. Look up towards the sky and picture your spine forming an imaginary 'U' shape.

4. As you exhale, round your spine and feel an imaginary string pull it towards to sky. Tuck your head down, towards your belly button and allow your hands and the tops of your feet to push you up from the ground.

5. On the next inhale repeat the entire sequence; allowing your belly to drop on the inhale and arch towards the sky on the exhale.

6. Repeat a total of 5 whole breaths.

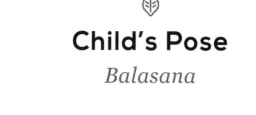

Child's Pose

Balasana

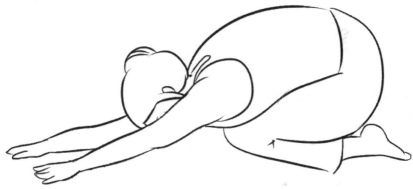

Again we revisit Child's Pose - the most restorative pose of them all, and one you will grow to love. As your yoga practice becomes more challenging and you feel stretched beyond your comfort zone, Child's Pose is the place you will return to. It's relaxing, calming, and brilliant for keeping your back healthy.

1. Settle yourself down onto the floor and get into a kneeling position. If your ankle or knees complain loudly, pop a folded-up blanket or small pillow under your bottom. If this doesn't do the trick, instead keep those feet close together but take your knees out wide to the side.

2. Now pop your arms in front of you, hands touching the ground.

3. Lean your body forward and down towards the ground as much as you can. Resist the urge to force yourself forward - just allow yourself to melt forward, releasing all tension from your body. Let your tummy rest either on your thigh, or between them, depending on which variation you are going for.

4. If you're already flexible, allow your forehead to rest on the floor. Pop a blanket underneath if this feels uncomfortable, and continue to let your body melt into the floor.

5. You can hold this pose for as long as you need. Why not try 5 breaths, or extend if you feel good in the pose?

These four postures are the perfect way to get a quick-fix of yoga into your life without having to adjust your busy schedule. And as a result, you should feel more relaxed, supple and de-stressed from everyday life.

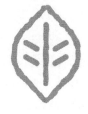

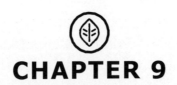

CHAPTER 9

Yoga & The Future:
Where To Go From Here

You should be feeling very proud of yourself - you've come so far! You've faced your fears and physical challenges, you've taken the time to find out what yoga is all about, and hopefully you've also started a yoga practice of your very own. I hope you've gotten comfortable with yoga and seen some really amazing benefits in your own health and happiness. You can now consider yourself a yogi!

So where do you go from here? How do you take your practice to the next level? Do you absolutely have to join a class with a teacher, or can you continue in the comfort of your own living room? How do you even know which teacher to choose?

This final chapter will address all of these issues, and show you how to take things to a whole new level and continue to improve those new-found skills.

Where Can I Go from Here?

The most effective way to take your practice to the next level isn't to read up on yogic philosophy or breathing techniques, although you can do these things if you so desire.

It's nailing the basics.

Go back through the book, look at the postures and consider how you could tweak them or progress further. There is always room for improvement - perhaps you'd like to touch your legs with your forehead when you do forward folds, maybe you'd like to touch the floor when you do triangle post, maybe you'd like to get those heels down when you unleash your downward facing dog. It really doesn't matter what it is, as long as it is important to you

Next pay attention to your breathing - are you listening to the rhythm of your breath? Are you breathing 'in time' with your postures? How could you improve?

Additionally, watch how you focus your attention as you practice. Are you able to zone in on your body and breath, or are you suffering from a severe case of money-brain, which chatters away with distracting information and steals your attention from where it could be? If so, ignore its attempts and allow your mind to quieten instead.

Do I Have to Join a Class?

This is one of the questions that I most commonly get asked, especially by curvier women who feel intimidated about the kind of people that they might find on the neighboring yoga mat. After all, they often don't want to put themselves 'out there' - they don't want to be judged and they don't want to come away feeling worse about themselves than before they went in. But they still want to take their practice to the next level, so feel frustrated and limited by their feelings.

I understand your concerns entirely. There's something about finding yourself in a room surrounded by athletic-looking individuals that will put fear into the most confident of us.

But there's really no need to worry. Yoga is inclusive, not exclusive, and your focus should be inward. Your only worry should be becoming the best possible version of yourself, whatever this might be. And you only get to that place by resisting the urge to compare yourself with those around you.

To answer your question, you don't have to join a class. If you did, then books like this one would not be possible. But it can be a wonderful supplement to your home practice to dip your toe into the world of yoga classes. Who knows - you might actually enjoy the social aspect and discover an inspiring teacher who can help you move towards achieving your health and fitness dreams.

How to Choose a Class

There are several things to bear in mind should you decide to give formal classes a go which will help you discover the perfect place for you to be.

You should look for a class that isn't too crowded, but isn't too quiet either. Both extremes are likely to make you feel more overwhelmed (and the latter is a bad sign when it comes to the quality of the classes).

The atmosphere in the room should be warm, friendly and welcoming, and most definitely not elitist or cold.

Finding the Right Teacher

Make sure you choose a teacher who is warm and supportive, and also helps you to feel completely at ease at all times. This isn't a place for frustrated corrections or angry words. Listen to your intuition on this one.

It also helps if your teacher is both comfortable with your curvier physique and understands that you will have unique needs. Feel free to ask a ton of questions, or even sit in on a class to see what it is like. Any teacher worth their two cents will be only too pleased to help you in any way that they can.

Needless to say, it's always a great idea to ask around in your local area to see which teachers are the most popular and why - doing this might help you to find some real gems!

Choosing Your Style

The approach in this book has been based around the hatha yoga style, which, as you have seen, is the most popular style of yoga and is perfect for beginners. However, this doesn't mean that you have to stick with this style as you move forward with your yoga practice.

Use the postures in this book as your foundation, and then take some time to figure out a style that's perfect for you - all of the styles vary in approach and intensity, so go for something that feels right for *you*. Sample a few classes or styles, either at home or in formal classes, see what is out there and then settle on the style that you love the best.

You don't win points for pushing yourself through a style that you hate - you simply defy the point of practicing yoga in the first place!

Don't be afraid to try some more advanced yoga moves, or head to a more advanced class when you feel ready - this might be just what you are looking for.

Most importantly, make sure that you fall in love with yoga. Don't force yourself through a practice (or class) that you despise, don't suffer a teacher who belittles you, be kind to yourself and accept your physical and mental limitations. And lastly, *ENJOY* your yoga practice.

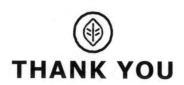

THANK YOU

Yoga is amazing for everyone no matter your size, age or gender. Don't 'buy in' to the adverts that try to convince you that you need to look in a certain way to practice, nor to get all of the incredible benefits that yoga offers. Everyone can do yoga, whether they are super-slender or more voluptuous.

As you have learned here, yoga will be your gateway to greater flexibility, strength, balance and health. And not only that, it will make you feel great on the inside too - you'll feel calmer, more focused, more confident and more in tune with your own thoughts and emotions. There's nothing quite like yoga in the entire world.

It is my hope that this book has given you everything you need to know about yoga in an accessible and easily understandable way that gently eases you into practice and helps you to grow. All you need to do now is put it all into action - incorporate yoga as a part of your daily life, boost your health with optimal nutrition, and take time to get outside and connect with those around you to unleash a sense of happiness and inner peace that you have only ever dreamed of.

I will leave you here, but be sure stay connected and in touch with the *Carma Books* community for more books on health and wellness, along with plenty of experiences and sharing of tips and knowledge on how to empower healing in your own life.

I hope that my guidance has helped you with your yoga journey, and that you will transform your life in just the way you wish. Good luck - and have fun!

A WORD FROM THE PUBLISHER

Hi, I'm Carmen, a holistic health geek with a passion for health, herbalism, natural remedies, as well as whole-food and plant-based lifestyles. After resolving various health issues I have struggled with for many years, I aim to inspire and help improve your health and longevity by sharing the tireless hours of research and valuable information I have discovered throughout my journey. Through the power of nutrition and lifestyle, with an evidence-based approach, I believe you can achieve your health and wellness goals.

If you enjoyed this book, I would love to hear how it has benefited you and invite you to leave a short review on Amazon - your valuable feedback is always appreciated!

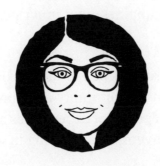

You are invited to to join our **Free Book Club** mailing list. Sign up via our website to receive **special offers** and *free for a limited time* Health & Wellness eBooks!

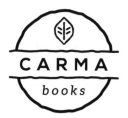

'A conscious approach to health & wellness'

carmabooks.com

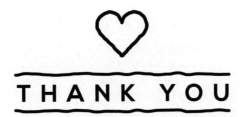

Printed in Great Britain
by Amazon